Less Stiff, Less Aches, No Sweat

Joint and Muscle Care for People who are Super Busy, Not So Bendy
or a Wee Bit Roundish

BLEU ANDERSEN, LMT

ISBN: 9798608917851

DEDICATION

This book is dedicated to all the clients who have given me purpose and drive.
Thank you for allowing me to assist in your recovery, contribute to your progress and
participate in your wellness.

CONTENTS

ACKNOWLEDGMENTS

I remain grateful to all those who have supported my efforts, practice, recovery and research

especially my dear Vince Beaudoin who encouraged and assisted daily

and, my classmate and fellow therapist, Anne Erickson, who asked me so very many times

"when are you going to write that book?".

INTRODUCTION

As a newly licensed massage therapist (LMT), finding myself struggling with osteoarthritis of the knee was quite daunting and discouraging. Months of swelling, fatigue, body-aches and limping left me with poor posture, limited range of motion and muscle weakness which in turn created weight gain, pain when performing my work, and numbness in my fingers while sleeping. I needed to regain ease, strength and flexibility and I needed to start where I was: stressed, stiff, sad and a bit scared.

Using my studies of myology, anatomy, neurology and shiatsu, I created short sessions to help me move toward recovery in stolen moments throughout the day. The simple movements eased my aches, allowed me to continue working and, in time, progress to full range of motion and recovery of strength.

I am feeling so much better and I want the same for you.

Break the cycle of aches and declining function while brewing coffee, watching TV or waiting for sleep. You will be delighted at the results.

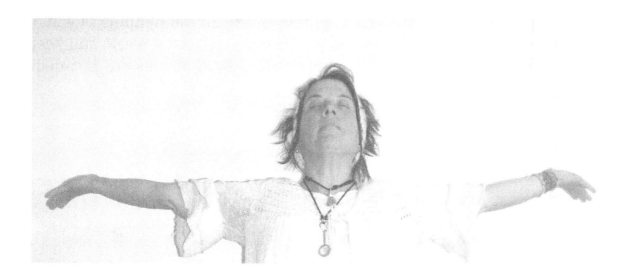

WHAT BRINGS YOU HERE?

Stretching and strengthening your muscles is an essential part of maintaining balance and range of motion as well as preventing injuries, aches and pains but so many of us simply don't have the time to go to the gym, or (gasp) hate yoga.

You probably spend a large part of your day in a fixed position due to occupation, commute, habit, hobby or injury. Your job may require repetitive tasks, contorted positions or heavy lifting. Over time, these will cause changes in posture and muscle function which can lead to aches, and limited range of motion. As the body tries to compensate and "keep it moving", more aches develop. Those aches, pains and limits, in turn, cause stress. Over time, these conditions lead to chronic pain, loss of function, sleep disturbances and other side effects of chronic stress such as poor digestion and depressed mood. Remember, stress is not just a mental experience; the chemicals which are released in the body affect muscles, organs, immunity and brain function.

I recommend therapeutic (not the same as a spa day) massage as regular maintenance to restore function, reduce stress, increase ease and prevent injuries, especially as the body ages, but it is what you are doing daily which will make the greatest difference.

Participate in your healing process and achieve the best possible results by sticking to this simple routine to loosen the joints, wake up sleepy muscles, increase lymph circulation, relax contracted muscles, increase flexibility and reduce stress.

I made this instructional as easy and as **brief** as possible because I know your time is precious. In fact, it may even be deceptively simplistic because, of course, much of this you have heard before, but the proof, as they say, is in the pudding. Read and practice the simple instructions, follow the program for at least a week, and keep a record of the positive changes you are experiencing so that you are inclined to continue with simple, sustainable, self-care.

UNDERSTANDING THE BODY

Years ago, I was watching a man who was having trouble starting his car. I knew he'd just had a gas pump installed so I suggested he pull his spark plugs and see if they needed scraping and gaping. They did. With clean plugs the car turned over.

I believe that if people understand what a spark plug does, they will be more likely to remember to do necessary maintenance. It is the same with body maintenance.

Beyond the obvious, why is breathing so important?

Your autonomic nervous system (ANS) controls lots of important things like organs, glands, circulation, pupil dilation... everything that goes on 'behind the scenes'. The ANS has two branches: sympathetic and parasympathetic.

The sympathetic branch ("fight or flight") is generally stuck in overdrive in modern society. Overstimulation leads to chronic stress and muscle tension. This does not feel good nor is it good for your health. You need to shut that down! It is meant for the rare adrenaline blast needed while fleeing or fighting for your life, but it has become the water in which we swim.

Luckily, there is something simple you can do for yourself every single day that will shut down that "fight or flight" mechanism AND it does not take time away from all the stuff on your To Do list..... correct breathing. No matter what else you are doing, you are breathing. Get determined to breathe right.

Deep, sustained, relaxed breathing stimulates the parasympathetic branch of the nervous system (the "rest and digest" portion) which decreases blood pressure, decreases adrenaline, decreases cortisol (the stress hormone) while increasing your immune response, digestion, endorphins (a natural pain killer) and serotonin (the happiness hormone). This will have a profound effect on your health, your experience of daily life as well as muscle tension.

In my practice, I have seen habitual shallow breathing result in diaphragms that were stiff from disuse and chronic neck pain due to contracted scalenes (which lift the top ribs when you take a deep breath).

Breath correctly during stretching but also throughout your day to keep your sympathetic nervous system on "standby".

Muscles need to move

Your muscles may not be zero-fat-camera-ready but they are worthy of being cherished and cared for. Not only do they help you move around, they also stabilize your joints, maintain your posture and generate heat.

When you contract your muscles with focus and effort, you not only reduce stiffness and increase strength, you also stimulate bone growth, increase lymph circulation (the cell sanitation service), and increase blood circulation (the cell meal delivery).

When you increase your flexibility through the stretches, you will experience increased balance, reduced the chance of injury, reduced pain, reduced stiffness and reduced pressure on your joints that can lead to or is presently causing inflammation. Remember, the suffix "-itis" simply means inflammation. Therefore, arthritis and bursitis are no more a life-sentence than laryngitis! If your "-itis" is sticking around for a long time, find an experienced LMT to help you lengthen the muscles around the joint, do these series daily and ask a nutritionist whether eliminating foods that cause inflammation will make a difference for you.

Lymph movement is just as important as blood flow

Lymph fluid is what removes toxins and waste from your cells and carries it to the filtering stations (nodes) where viruses, bacteria and cancer cells are separated out and discarded. It is also an essential part of your immune response because it delivers white blood cells which defend the body against infection. Stagnation reduces your immune response and can lead to swelling, soreness and disease.

Look at it this way, if you bagged up your garbage but left it in the kitchen how long would that take to get nasty? What if you stopped taking out the garbage all together and it has been accumulating for months? Years? Move your Lymph!

How? The muscle contractions in the following series increase this vital lymph circulation. The stretches create long, relaxed muscles which allow lymph to flow freely. Something else you can do to increase circulation of lymphatic fluid is fluid-moving or lymphatic massage from a licensed therapist. (Please, let your spouse off the hook, pry open your wallet and hire a professional LMT for best results). Other things you can look into for healthy lymph circulation are dry-brushing, brisk walks, rebounding or (my least favorite of all) a cold rinse after a hot shower. BRRR!

Grease the Joints

If you let your car sit in the garage for a few years, the wheels will have a really hard time rolling until you redistribute the grease in wheel bearings and axels. In a similar way, free-moving joints in the body are wrapped with fluid filled capsules. Movement of the joints warm and distribute these fluids making it easier for you to move. That is why the series includes circular movements of the joints.

Fascia Restrictions are Quite Common

There is a connective tissue in your body called fascia. It is like a microscopic disorganized spider web. It surrounds your ever cell, every fiber, every organ, and every bone. It is a wonderful stabilizing force, however, when you have an injury it can become a bit overzealous in its job. Fascial restrictions can severely limit your range of motion after surgery, broken bones or after recovery from something like bursitis. Stretching every day can break up these restrictions over time. For faster results, hire an LMT experienced in MFR (myo-fascial release).

The Subtle Channels

There are 12 very subtle channels, called meridians, which act as a bridge between your body's physical experience and the non-physical aspects of your being such as emotions, will, mind and spiritual expression.

Eastern medicine has been addressing meridian health for thousands of years through modalities like acupuncture and shiatsu, although when it comes to scientific proof, the meridians have been more elusive than the Higgs Boson. However, in the 1960's Bon Han Kim was able track the physical presence of these channels using a stain. The experiment was later validated by Dr. Kwang-Sup Soh.

Like lymph and blood vessels, these channels pass throughout the body's muscles, joints and organs and so removing blockages to maintain flow is utterly important. Traditionally, this is accomplished by a series of poses called Makka Ho stretches which require lots of flexibility. That is why I developed the Weekend Series. Stretch and flow is easily and effectively accomplished with these movements and you will notice right away.

BREATHING DEEP AND WIDE

The right kind of breathing activates relaxation responses in the nervous system as well as delivers much needed oxygen…. Both impact the muscles. It is absolutely essential that you learn how to breathe correctly and practice correct breathing while you are stretching or performing isometric contractions.

Do it now with me…..

Through your nose, start a long slow inhale deep in the belly. Use your diaphragm.

Continue inhale until the chest widens.

Continue inhale until the shoulders rise just a bit.

Hold for one second.

Slowly, blow out through your mouth. (Sigh if you like.)

Repeat completely and patiently 4 times. (Don't cheat. It takes only one minute!)

Notice the subtle difference this makes.

When you practice the exercises in this book, breathe deep and wide for the best results. If you are like many people, you will be tempted to hold your breath when making an effort or to breath in a shallow manner. Focus on changing that habit.

In fact, if you could get into the habit of long, slow, deep breaths throughout the day, your body will reward you with increased calm and clarity even when faced with a confrontational customer, bad news from the doctor, family drama or particularly difficult work situation.

STRETCH PROPERLY

Long, relaxed muscles are the goal. It will increase your range of motion, prevent aches and keep nerves from being pinched. Stretching correctly is essential.

First of all, forget the bouncing you were taught in school. Reaching for your toes and bouncing sends the wrong message to the brain. Too fast of a stretch will cause the muscle to contract.

Instead, after a few calming breaths, move into the stretch position, allow gravity to do the work as you continue to breath deep and wide. Long, slow breaths activate the parasympathetic nervous system which allows muscles to relax. Consistent and sustained stretch on the tendons (which attach muscle to bone) sends a message to the brain that the muscle needs to lengthen and that is how you get your stretch. Stretching every day accomplishes 'muscle re-education' which is exactly what it sounds like. Muscles form habits that can be broken by consistent repetition over a period of time just like when you are house-training your new rescue pup.

It is gravity, breath, time and repetition which will yield the best results. But don't worry, the series in this book will slide seamlessly into the pauses of your day and will not cause the kind of disturbance that makes you want to skip a day in the way that the dread of changing clothing and driving to the gym does.

I realize it all sounds much too simple BUT, if you do the series every day, you will see progress and restoration. Don't give up before you begin.

IS IT PAIN OR JUST DISCOMFORT?

When doing the movements in these series, it is normal and expected to have discomfort and even aches in areas which have been restricted for a long while.

Do not, however, do anything which causes pain or cramping.

What is the difference?

Discomfort is simply "oh, I feel that". There is no alarm, no retreat, just awareness. This is normal and desirable because these places are in need of care and change.

Ache is what you feel when lifting something which is too heavy. You may groan or even say "wow". You hesitate, focus and proceed with caution. When you feel an ache during one the movements in these series, pause and take extra time for long, deep, easy breathing. Do not push beyond your present limitation. Notice that ease comes after a few long breaths. If you do the movements regularly, you will notice that those aches are much improved or absent.

Pain, on the other hand, is like dropping a cinderblock on your foot; there is an immediate shock and recoil. If you feel pain during the series, stop and back up to a place where there is no pain nor cramping. Do not, however, omit the movement from your routine unless directed by your doctor. Places of pain or cramping are desperately in need of change. Back up, pause, breath and approach the threshold slowly. Remain at the threshold, and breath. Just as with aches, you will notice more ease come with breathing and repetition over a period of time. For returning issues, find an excellent massage therapist who can do postural assessment, treatment and suggest changes that will further your goals.

WHAT IS ISOMETRIC?

Isometric simply means that the length of the muscle remains the same; the bones and joints do not move. When you see some dude doing "The Gun Show" in the mirror THAT'S an isometric contraction. Do not become discouraged if it takes some practice to get the targeted muscle to respond fully. Many muscles are sleepy and weak from not being used. Visualize success clearly (to rebuild neural pathways) until you achieve success.

Be aware of compensation that can accompany weakened muscle response. This means that the muscles surrounding the targeted muscle are doing the work. Compensation happens quite often as muscles become tired and our posture progressively grows more poor.

When we routinely do not engage a muscle, the nerve-messages stop being delivered….. kind of like a postal route being re-routed. Visualization re-establishes the delivery route and eventually the "driver" gets through. I learned this from a woman who was told she'd be unable to walk for the rest of her life by her doctors. She spent months visualizing movement of the target muscles and today, after years of consistent effort, walks as well as she ever did. So, if the target muscle is not engaging when you tell it, visualize, focus and try again and again until you succeed. You can always show your LMT who can assess which muscles are compensating and help you address any fascial restrictions keeping you from progressing.

Benefits of Isometric Contractions:

1. Relief from aches and limited range of motion. When muscles are partially contracted at all times, a full contraction is often followed by complete release.

2. Release of the opposing muscles. Contracting a muscle fully automatically causes the opposing muscles to release. It is hardwired that way. Each joint is controlled by two opposing sets of muscles. In order to work together smoothly, when one side contracts the other side relaxes to allow the movement.

3. Muscle contractions move lymph.

CHECK IN / CHECK OUT

Take a moment to remind yourself that this is only a few minutes out of your day. Everything can wait for this short time while you do important repairs and care.

Before you begin any session, calmly take inventory of your body, mind and emotions. Where are the places that feel achy or stiff? Scan your head, neck, shoulders, wrists, back, legs, and ankles.

What is on your mind? Are you stressed? Are you worried? Is your breathing shallow? Are you twitchy?

Enjoy a few minutes of silence, or put on some music if you wish or a program that you ENJOY! Something light and soothing is good medicine so please forgo the nightly news. If you have children who want your attention, get them involved. The sooner they learn body care, the less likely they will suffer an injury when playing sports, and if they keep it up they will age much more gracefully.

After checking in with your body, focus on your first deep, full breath. Be present and conscious. Give yourself this time as a gift of brief minutes and simple movements; an investment in your wellness, recovery and ease.

As you move through the series, if your mind tries to make lists or rush the process or insists on worry, stop and re-focus on your breathing. It may help to count seconds: breath in to the count of 6, pause, breath out to the count of 6, pause, etc.

And then, and this is <u>equally</u> important, at the very end take inventory again.

Make note of the positive changes that will inspire you to continue.

GET STARTED

The remaining chapters are the short series of movements you can scatter throughout your day without losing precious time from your busy schedule. Tear out the 'quick lists' to place for easy access. I strongly suggest you keep a record of the benefits that you notice so that you are prompted to keep the good times rolling.

Feel better.....

Day	Notes
1	
2	
3	
4	
5	
6	
7	

SNOOZE BUTTON SERIES - 5 minutes

This is a great excuse to stay in bed for a few extra minutes! Use this time to gently warm up your joints and muscles before you begin your day.

Making circles with your joints warms the synovial fluid inside of each joint capsule. Gentle stretches of the joints ease the pressure caused by stiff muscles and can prevent aches before they even begin.

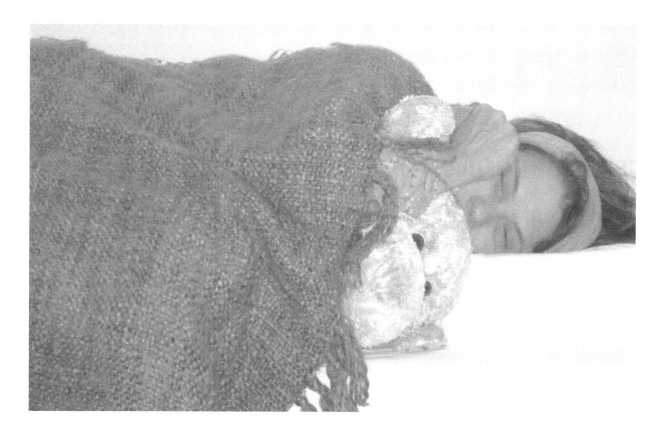

ANKLES AND WRIST CIRCLES

Trace circles with your wrists then your ankles.
5 to 12 times clockwise then counterclockwise.

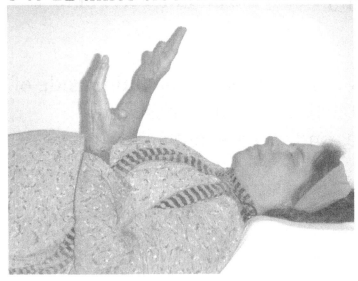

FINGER AND THUMB CIRCLES

Gently pull your fingertip.
Trace 5 to 12 small circles.
Repeat for all fingers and thumbs.

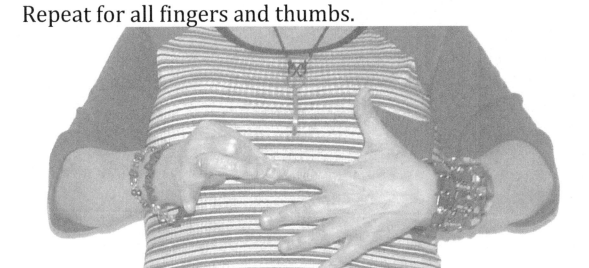

SPINAL TWIST

Turn your head to the right.
Rest your right arm on the bed.
Cross your right leg over the body.
Breath long and deep 3 to 5 times.
Repeat for the other side.

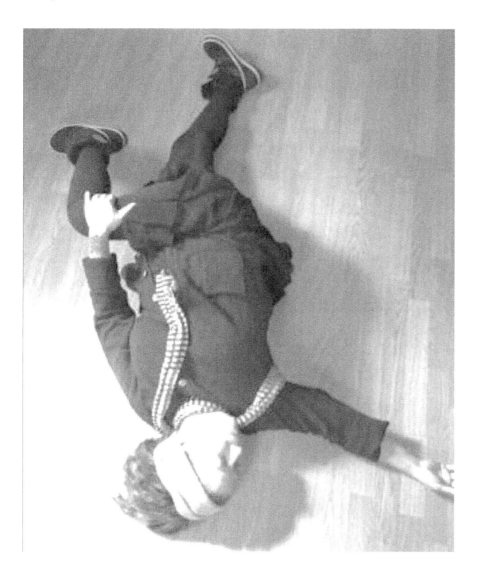

HIP AND KNEE STRETCH

Take 3 to 5 long deep breaths at each position.
With knee straight, use a scarf to pull toes toward face.
Lower the leg to the side (stretch inner thigh and knee)
Cross leg over the body (stretch outer thigh and knee)
Repeat for the other leg.

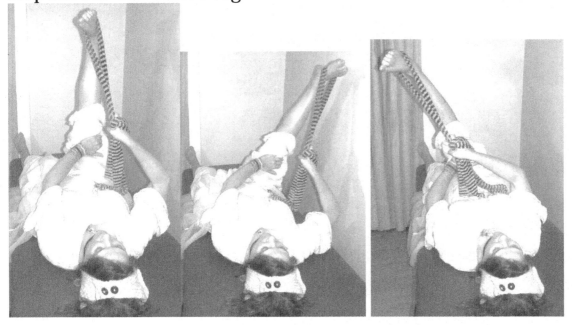

Look at the progress I have made! My knees feel much better.

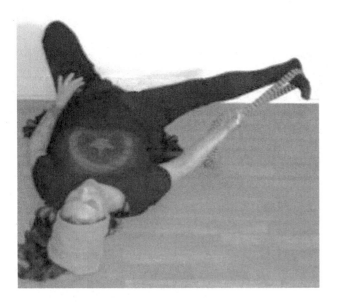

BELLY STRETCH

Turn onto your belly.
Rest on your elbows (stretch abdomen)
Look up. Breathe deeply 3 to 5 times.

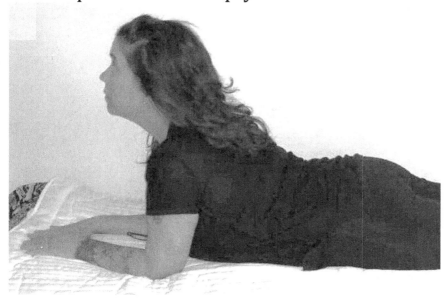

If able, rise up on your hands with hips on the bed. Breathe.

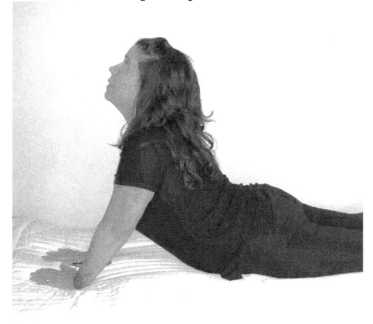

HIPS, SHOULDERS, UPPER BACK STRETCH

With knees apart, sit on your heels.
Stretch arms overhead. Breathe deeply 3 to 5 times.

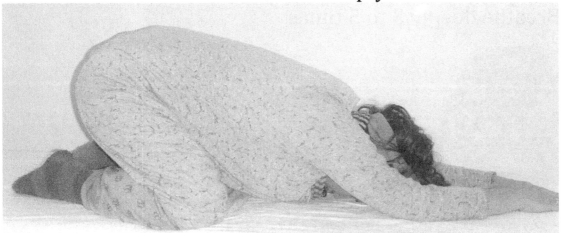

A word of encouragement:
When I first started, I could barely bend my knees or expand my hips. It was quite uncomfortable but I continued to work within my limits consistently and saw progress over time.

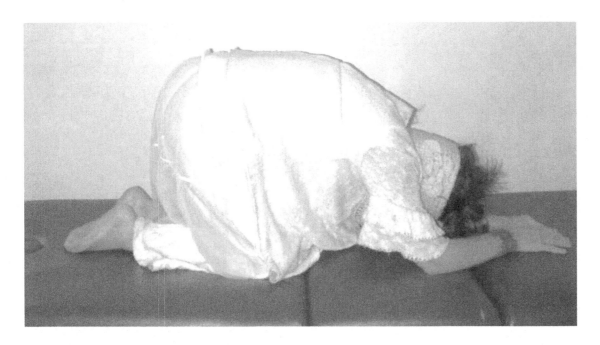

NECK CIRCLES

Sit up and make 5 to 12 little circles with your neck.
Clockwise and then counterclockwise.
Shake your head "no" 12 times, then nod up and down 12 times.

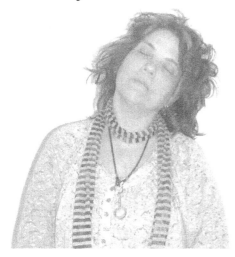

SHOULDER ROLLS

Make 5 to 12 circles with your shoulders, forward then back.

(Yes, I sleep with a scarf and hat sometimes. My house is cold.)

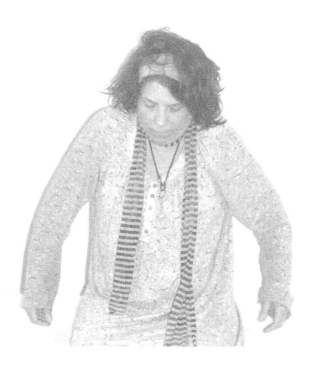

EYE CIRCLES

Surprise! Your eyes have muscles that need unstiffening. Move your hand as if pointing to the numbers on a big clock. Have your eyes follow your hand in circles 5 to 12 times. Clockwise and then counterclockwise.

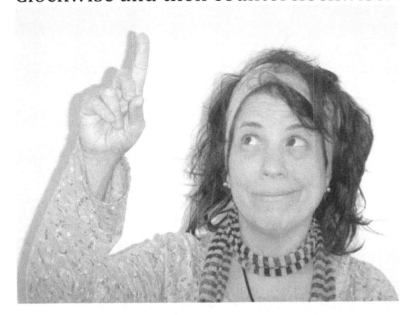

You are ready to get dressed and start your coffee pot.

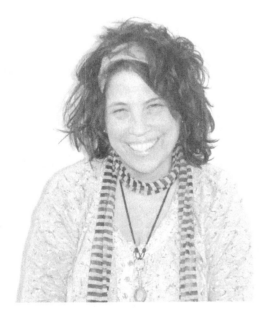

SNOOZE BUTTON SERIES

QUICK LIST (Tear out and place in your bedroom.)

1. Wrist circles

2. Ankle circles

3. Finger and thumb circles

4. Spine twist

5. Hip and knee stretches (3)

6. Belly stretch

7. Hip/Shoulder/Upper Back

8. Neck circles

9. Shoulder rolls

10. Eye circles

This page intentionally left blank.

COFFEE POT SERIES - 3 minutes

As I stand at the counter waiting for my coffee brew, I am still half asleep. Being good for little else during those few minutes, I use the time to stretch and strengthen my ankles and hips.

Our toes and ankles tend to become compressed and immobile from the shoes that we wear, leading to chronic ankle and knee troubles. Simple daily stretches can prevent troubles and ease aches. Whenever possible, walk barefoot. To prevent slipping, try gripper socks or water shoes (shown below). Although they are popular, I've seen slides, crocs and flip-flops cause lots of problems with my clients' legs because the foot is constantly (and unconsciously) flexed to keep the shoe on.

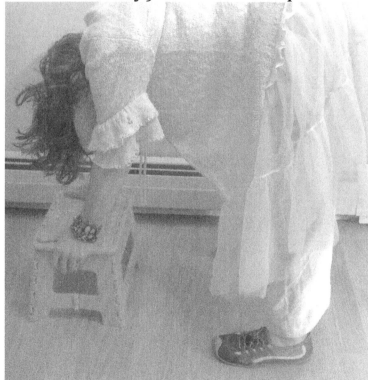

TOE STRETCH

Top of big toe on the floor in front (stretch toes)
Roll slightly to stretch smaller toes.
Hold for 1 to 2 breaths.
Repeat on other side.

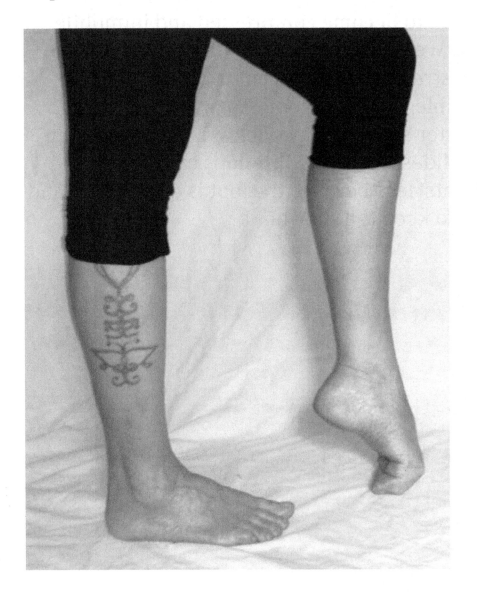

FRONT OF ANKLE STRETCH

Top of toes on floor behind you. (stretch front of ankle)
Hold for 1 to 2 breaths.
Repeat on other side.

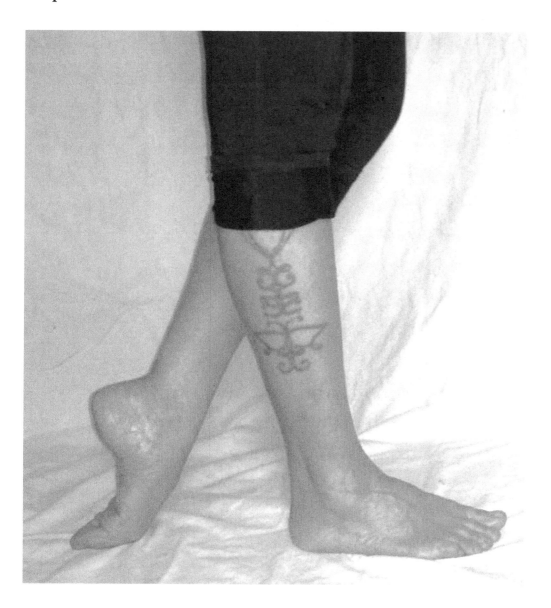

INSTEP STRETCH

Bottom of your toes behind (stretch the instep)
Hold for 1 to 2 breaths.
Repeat on other side.

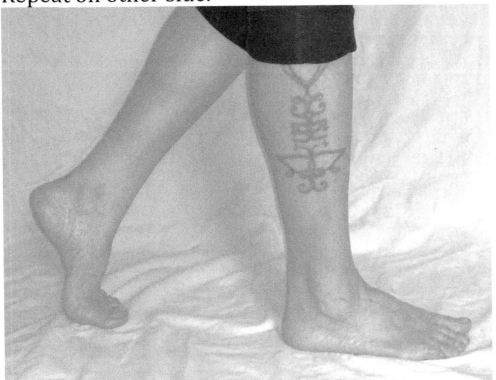

(In case you are wondering, my tattoo is of my grandmother's name. Tilt your head to the left. Her name was Grace.)

CALF STRETCH

Straighten rear knee, heel on the floor.
Bend forward knee to stretch calf.
Hold for 2 to 3 breaths.
Repeat on other side.

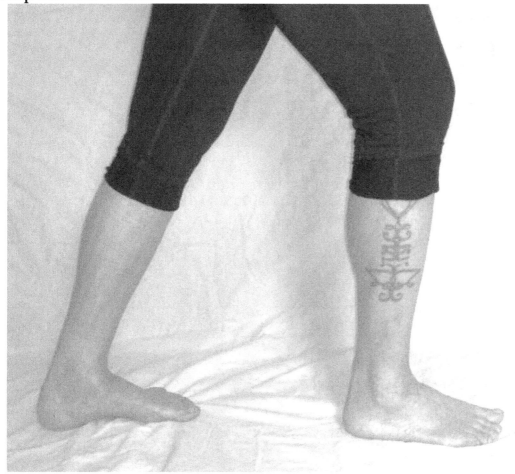

ACHILLES STRETCH

Heels on floor, bend both knees (stretch Achilles tendon)
Hold for 2 to 3 breaths.
Repeat for other side.

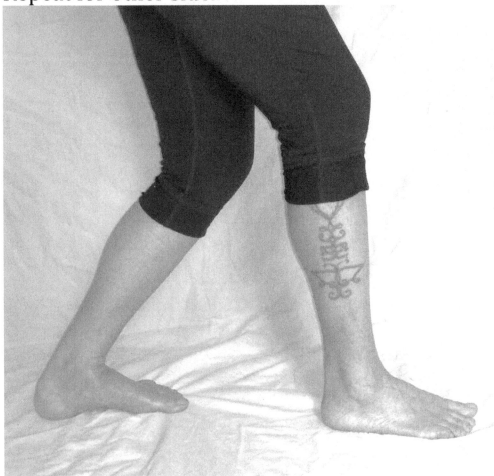

ANKLE STRETCH

Pinky toe on floor (stretch outer ankle)
Big toe on floor (stretch inner ankle)
Repeat on the other side.

Note: you may feel this in your knee as well.

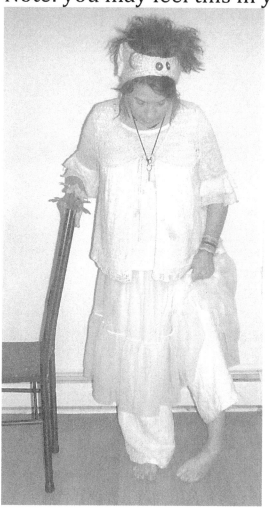 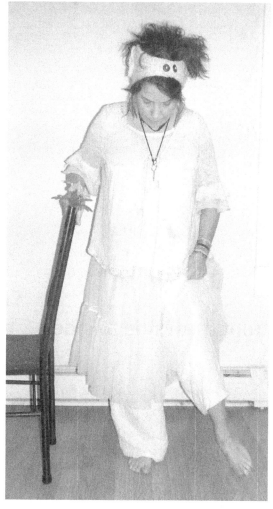

HIP SOCKET CIRCLES

Make 10 or 12 large circles with each leg.

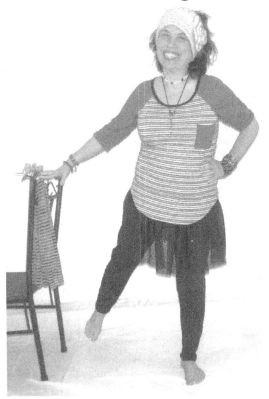

"Wag" each foot from side to side 12 times.

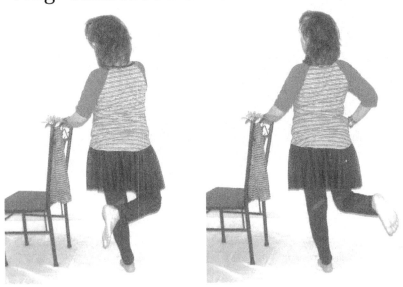

STRENGTHEN LEGS

Rise up on your toes 10 to 15 times (feel in calves)

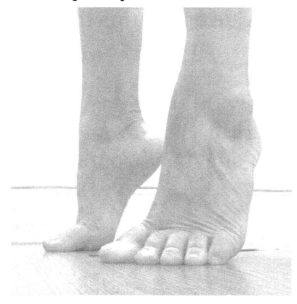

Finish with 20 to 30 mini-squats (feel in thighs)
(Believe me, I hate squats as much as you but when my legs got super shaky on the stairs I figured it was better to suffer for 30 seconds every morning than to take a tumble.)

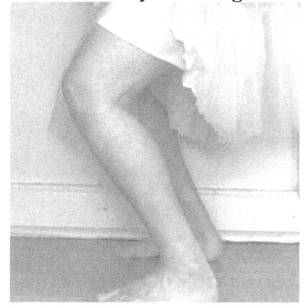

COFFEE TIME!!

Remember to drink an equal amount of water for every caffeinated (or alcoholic) beverage you indulge in during the day. I don't do this....but you should. Hahahha.

Just kidding....mostly.   Sometimes I actually DO try to drink enough Berkey filtered water but not nearly as often as I should. Water is the closest thing we have to the Fountain of Youth.

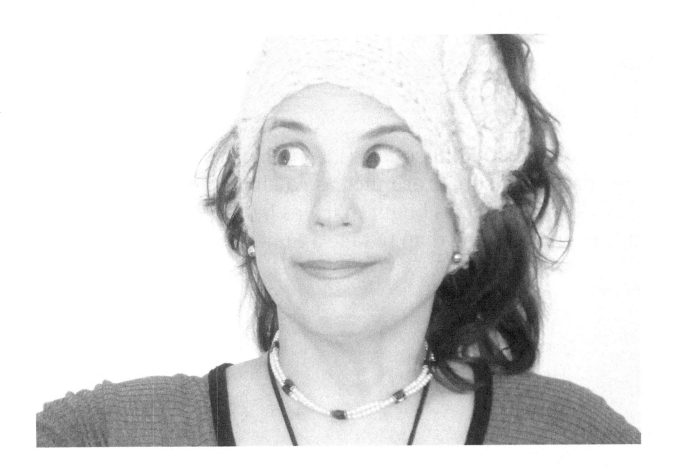

COFFEE POT SERIES

QUICK LIST (Tear out and place in your kitchen.)

1. Toe Top Stretch
2. Foot Top Stretch
3. Instep Stretch
4. Calf Stretch
5. Achilles Stretch
6. Ankle Side Stretches (2)
7. Leg Circles
8. Leg "Wag"
9. Tippy Toes
10. Aaaargh. Squats!

This page intentionally left blank.

<u>BREAK TIME SERIES - 5 minutes</u>

Take a short break during the day especially if you are in a fixed position (such as driving or keyboarding) or perform the same task repeatedly (like contractors or musicians).

These stretches can maintain the muscles in a long, relaxed state to prevent pain at the shoulders, aches at the elbows, tingling at the fingers or sciatic nerve irritation.

Breathing is key. Do not rush.

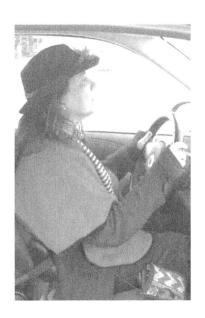 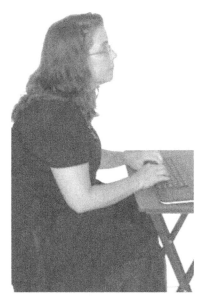 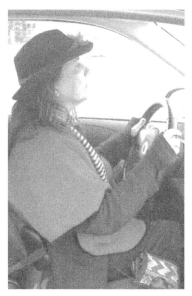

NECK AND SHOULDER STRETCH

Sit comfortably. Place your left hand under your thigh.
Drop head to the right with nose facing forward. Breath 3 or 4x.

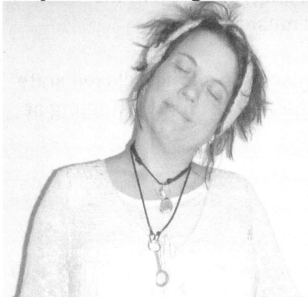

Rotate head so that nose is toward ceiling. Breath 3 or 4 times.

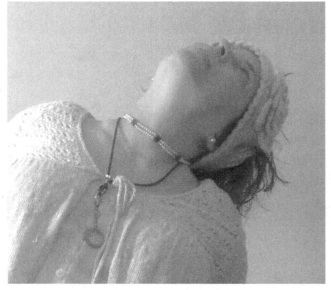

Rotate head like you are sniffing your right shoulder. Breathe.
(not pictured)

Repeat 3 positions for other side.

DIGITS AND WRIST STRETCH

Turn your left palm up, elbow straight.
Use your right hand to pull your thumb. Breath.
Repeat with each finger. Pause and breathe for each.
Repeat with other hand.

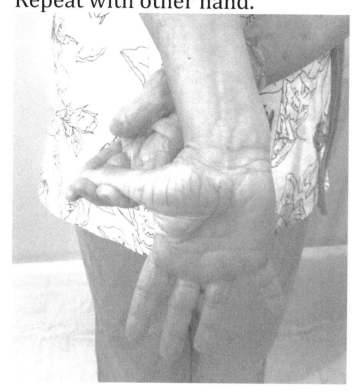

Stretch back of wrist with fingers curled and elbow straight.

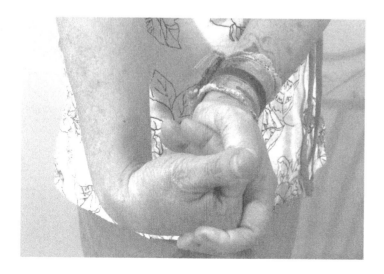

SHOULDER PRESS AND SPIN

Sit in a chair for balance.
Spread arms and fingers, press wrists back.
Arch back and squeeze shoulders together.
Hold 5 -10 seconds and repeat.

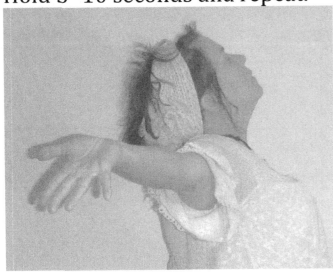

Turn your palms toward the ceiling.
Rotate both arms forward until palm faces behind.
Repeat 5 to 12 times.

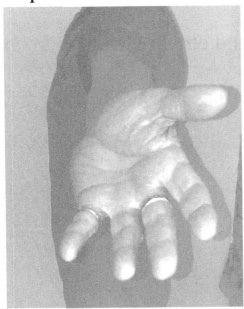 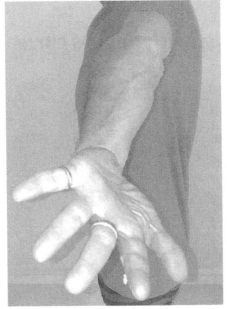

SCIATIC NERVE CARE

Place left ankle on right knee.
Push left knee down gently and hold right ankle.
With straight back, lean forward. Breath 3 to 4 times.

Cross left leg over right leg.
With straight back, pull knee toward chest. Breath 3 times.
Repeat on the other side.

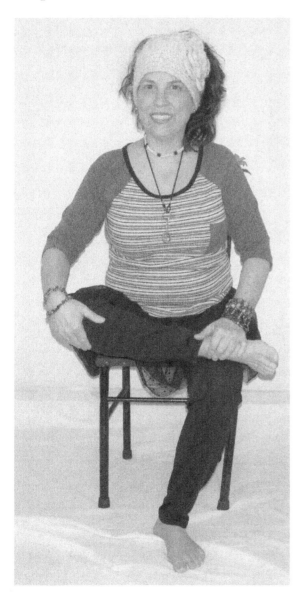
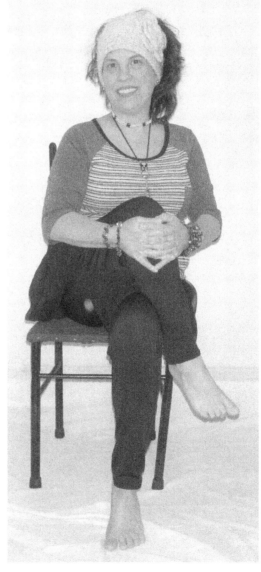

This page intentionally left blank.

BREAK TIME SERIES

QUICK LIST (Tear out and take to work.)

1. Neck/Shoulder Stretches
    a. Side
    b. Face Up
    c. Face Down
2. Thumb Stretches
3. Finger Stretches
4. Back of Wrist Stretch
5. Shoulder Press
6. Shoulder Spin
7. Sciatic Nerve Care
    a. Ankle to Knee
    b. Knee over Knee

This page intentionally left blank.

DINNER PREP SERIES - 10 minutes

Giving yourself a few minutes to shake off the day is good medicine. These stretches are especially good for people who have knee pain, back aches or fatigue. You can do this while your dinner is cooking.

Especially, do not skimp on your spine time! Contracted muscles put pressure on the tiny joints that make up the spine...joints where your nerves exit the spinal column on their way towards to your limbs and organs. That pressure can irritate those tiny joint capsules and lead to inflammation. No Bueno!

Life is busy, I understand, but injury that keeps you out of work or steals your joy is worth preventing. Use a chair for balance if needed.

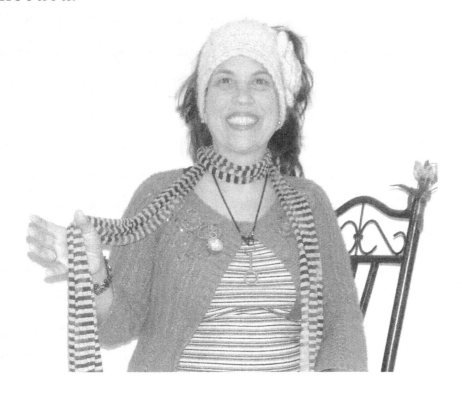

SIDE BODY STRETCH

Place your feet wide with right arm behind your back.
Turn your right toe in and stick your right hip out.
Feel a stretch at the right hip, left knee and front of shoulder.
Lean to your left. Breathe.
Bend your left knee to increase stretch.
Breathe 3 to 5 times.

Lift your arm for a torso stretch. Breathe 2 or 3 times.
Repeat on the other side.

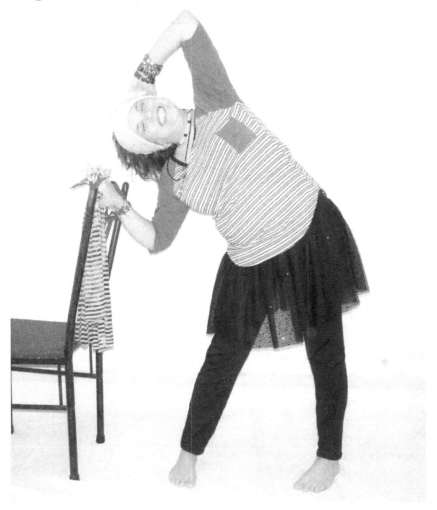

ABDOMINAL STRETCH

Place hands behind your back or hold a chair for balance.
Arch back with head up (stretch abs). Breathe 3 to 5 times.

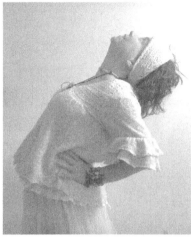

Lean slightly left. Breathe 2 or 3 times.
Return to center.
Lean slightly right. Breath 2 or 3 times.

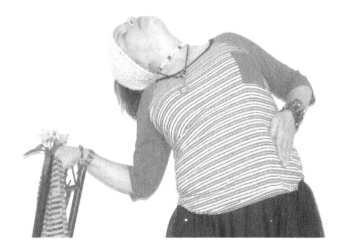

THIGH AND HIP STRETCH

If you cannot reach your ankle, use a scarf.
Bend knee (stretch thigh).
Arch back (stretch front of hip). Breath 3 to 5 times.

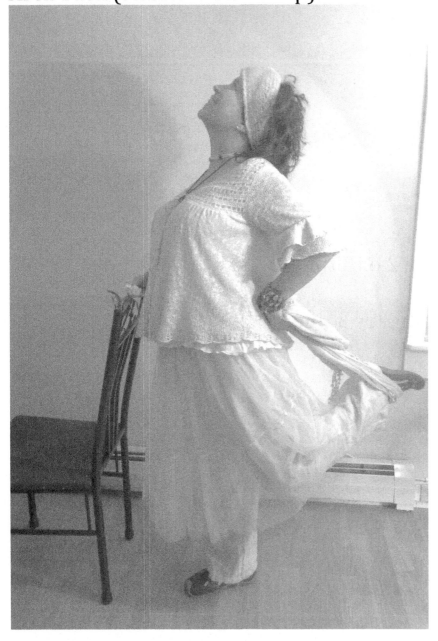

LEGS AND LOWER BACK STRETCH

Point toes slightly inward.
Bend forward with straight knees and straight back.
Push your bottom back until you feel lower leg stretch. Breathe.

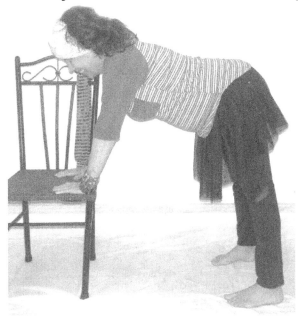

Keep knees straight. Bend forward to stretch buttocks. Breathe.

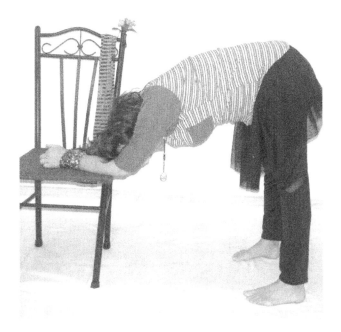

UPPER BACK STRETCH

Bend knees and hang from middle back. Breathe 2 or 3 times.

Straighten a bit, stretch between shoulder blades. Breath 2 or 3x.

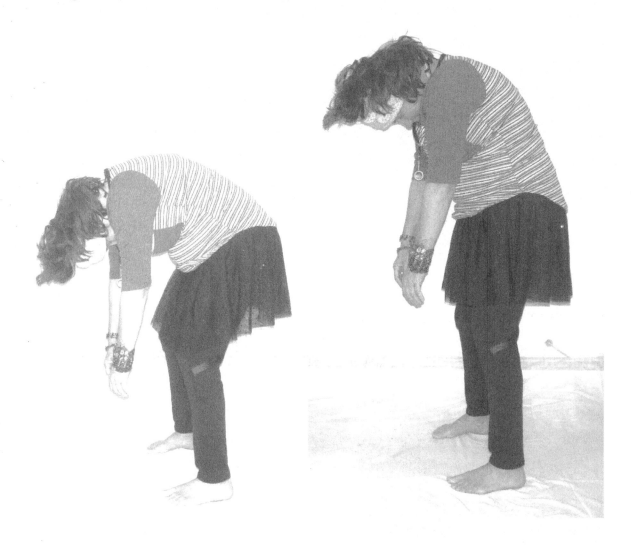

DINNER PREP SERIES

QUICK LIST (Tear out and place in your kitchen.)

1. Side Body Stretch
2. Abdominal Stretch
   a. Midline
   b. Off center, left and right
3. Front Thigh/Hip Stretch
4. Leg/Glute Stretch
5. Lower/Upper Back Stretch

This page intentionally left blank.

<u>TV TIME SERIES - 5 minutes</u>

Full contraction of muscles re-builds nerve pathways, moves lymph, and makes relaxation possible for the target muscle and the opposing muscle.

Be sure to contract the target muscle with ALL your effort and focus for 10 to 20 seconds. These contractions are isometric meaning bones remain in the same place throughout the effort.

You won't look like a body builder after but you will feel better.

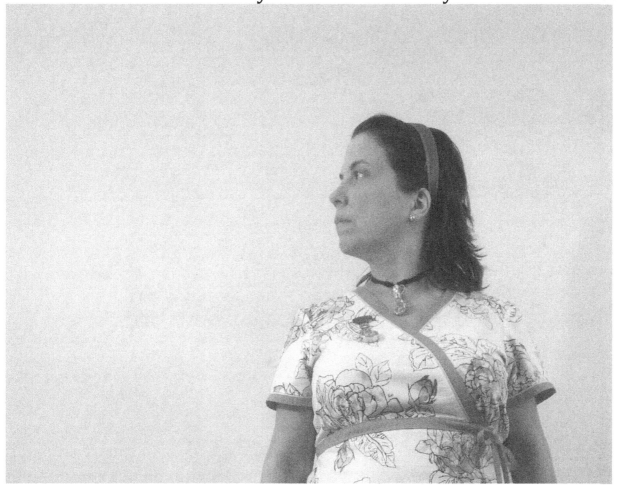

FRONT OF LEG CONTRACTION

With focused effort, simultaneously:
Flex your foot
Straighten your leg forcefully
Lift your leg an inch off the chair
Hold for 10 to 20 seconds

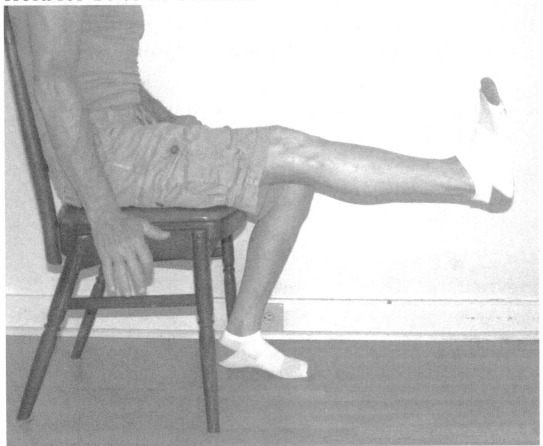

SHOULDER BLADE CONTRACTIONS

With focused effort, simultaneously:
Straighten your back
Press your elbows toward your spine forcefully
Hold for 10-20 seconds

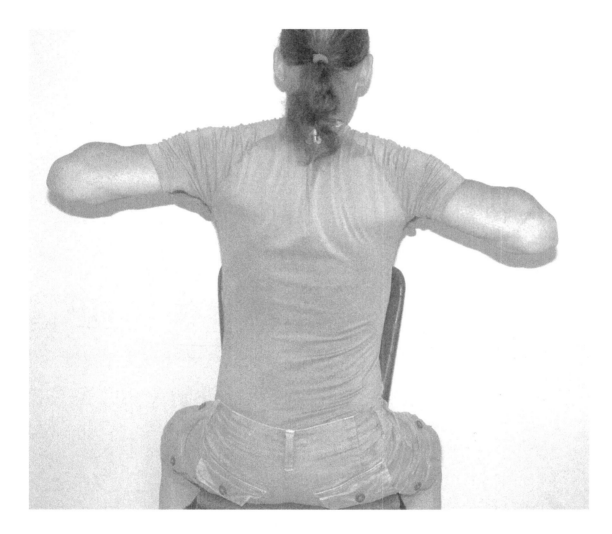

HARD SHRUG

With focused effort, simultaneously:
Squeeze your shoulders to your ears
Press your neck back (don't tilt head up)
Hold for 10-20 seconds

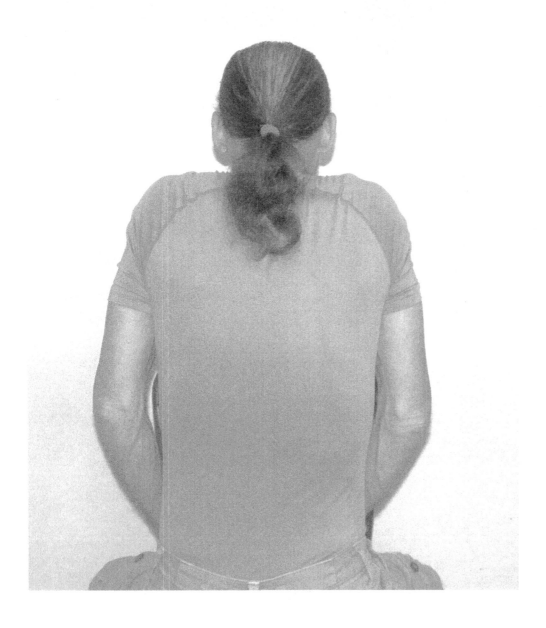

LENGTHEN THE NECK

With focused effort, simultaneously:
Straighten your arms
Press elbows into the body
Reach to the ground with your hands
Reach for the ceiling with your head
Hold for 10-20 seconds

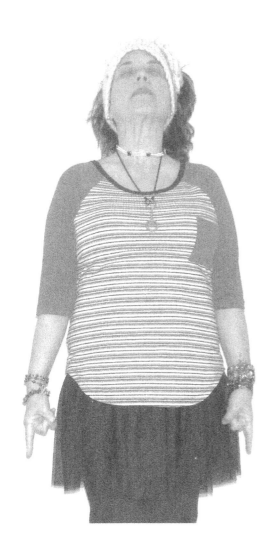

CONTRACT THE CHEST

With focused effort, simultaneously:
Straighten your back
Cross arms
Reach for the opposite walls forcefully
Hold for 10-20 seconds

Place the other arm on top, and repeat

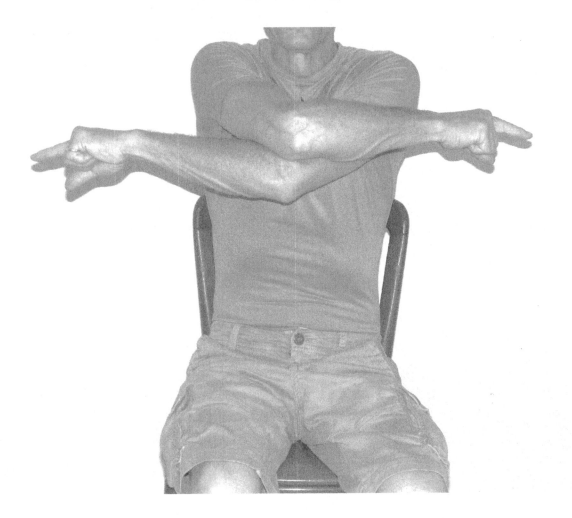

BICEPS AND BACK CONTRACTION

With focused effort, simultaneously:
Pull up on your thighs
Resist the pull with your legs and back
Hold for 10-20 seconds

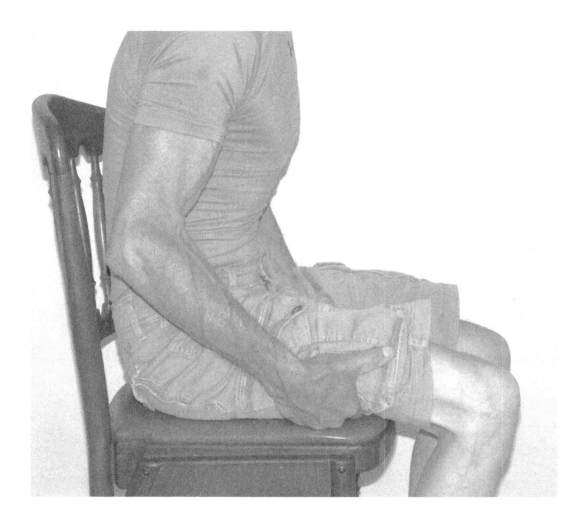

TRICEP AND AB CONTRACTION

With focused effort, simultaneously:
Press down on your thighs
Resist the press with your abdomen
Hold for 10-20 seconds

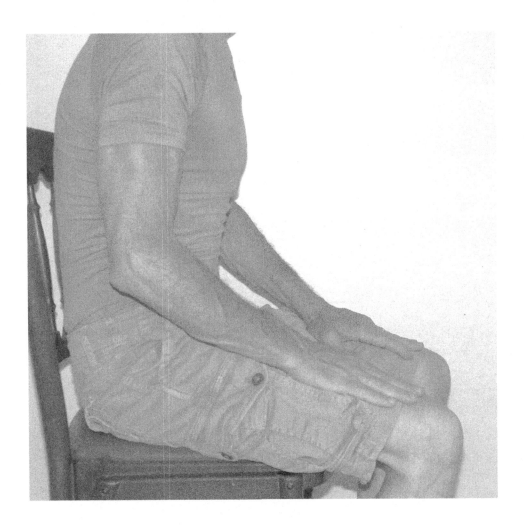

BACK NECK CONTRACTION

With focused effort, simultaneously:
Press your head back into the spine forcefully
Jut your chin to the ceiling
Roll shoulders back
Hold for 10-20 seconds

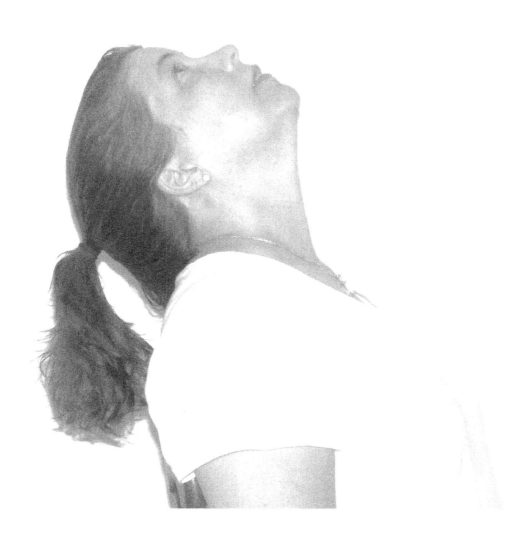

FRONT NECK CONTRACTION

With focused effort, simultaneously:
Press your chin into your chest forcefully
Roll shoulders forward
Hold for 10-20 seconds

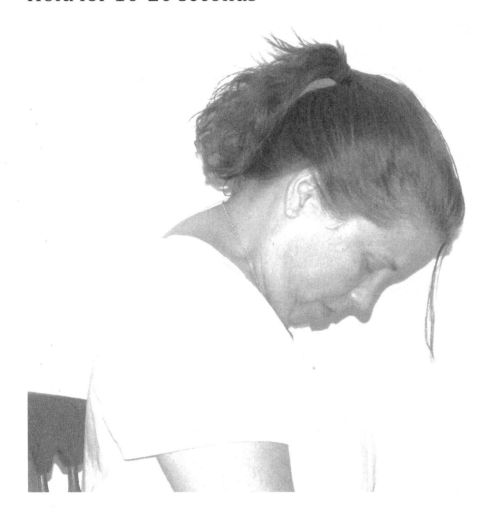

CHIN TO SHOULDER

With focused effort, simultaneously:
Turn your head as far right as possible
Press shoulders down
Hold for 10-20 seconds
Repeat for the other side

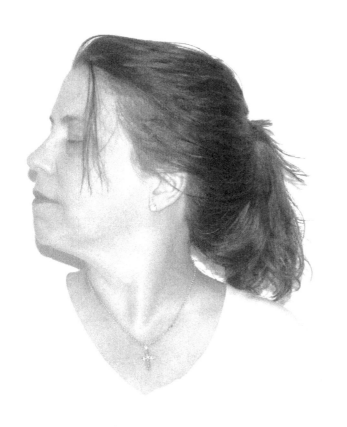

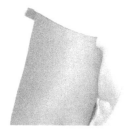

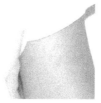

This page intentionally left blank.

TV TIME SERIES

QUICK LIST (Tear out and place near your television.)

1.   Front of Leg
2.   Shoulder blades
3.   Hard shrug
4.   Lengthen the Neck
5.   Contract the Chest
6.   Biceps and Back Contraction
7.   Tricep and Ab Contraction
8.   Back of Neck Contraction
9.   Front of Neck Contraction
10. Chin to Shoulder

64

This page intentionally left blank.

<u>BED TIME SERIES - 5 minutes</u>

Taking a few minutes before sleep to fully contract muscles will leave you feeling relaxed. It is a great way to shake off the day and rest well.

When you first are doing these exercises, it may take a few tries to get the target muscle to respond. That is normal. The neural connection to the muscle will get stronger. Until then, visualize the contraction and keep trying.

Incidentally, this is a great way to spend time when you are stuck in bed. Keep your blood moving and your muscles warm!

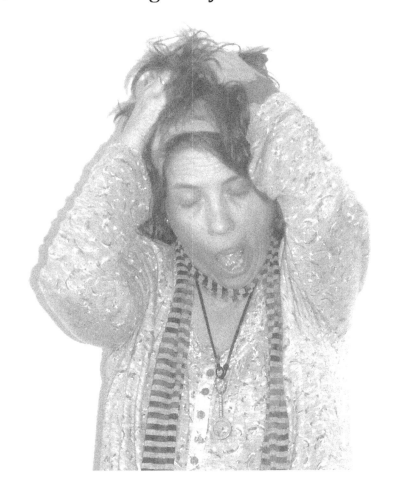

STRENGTHEN ANKLES

With focused effort,
Curl your toes toward your face. Hold for 10 to 20 seconds.
Turn your ankles outward. Hold for 10 to 20 seconds.
Turn your ankles inward. Hold for 10 to 20 seconds.
Point your toes. Hold for 10 to 20 seconds.

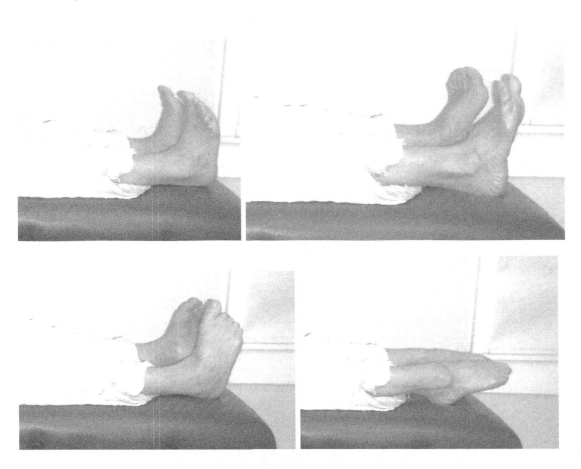

ALL OVER CONTRACTIONS

With focused effort, contract, and hold each for 10-20 seconds.

All muscles in the front of the leg (repeat other side)
All muscles in the back of the leg (repeat other side)
All muscles of hand and arm (repeat other side)
Abdominal muscles
Back muscles
Press head into the mattress

Release and relax all muscles
Draw in breath until your belly, chest and shoulders are full
Hold for 3 seconds
Blow all air out, squeeze out the last bit with your belly
Remain empty for 3 seconds and repeat cycle 3 or more times.

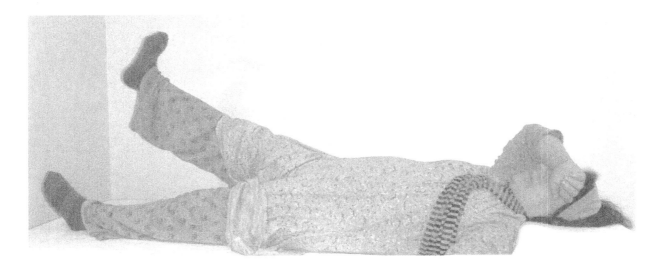

Sweet dreams.

This page intentionally left blank.

<u>**WEEKEND SERIES - 20 minutes**</u>

Flow from one stretch to the next. Pause at each stretch and breathe deeply as many times as needed to create ease. Use a chair or scarf if needed.

Subtle channels running throughout the body have been documented by Eastern medicine for centuries. These meridians are essential for health of the body, mind and spirit. Treatment of the meridians is the purpose of acupuncture and shiatsu. This movement series will create flow through all the meridians in order. The results will speak for themselves.

As always, do only what you are able. Focus on where <u>you</u> are feeling the stretch, not the ability of demonstration models. Even if you are not flexible, do what you can to create a relaxed, easy feeling in your body and mind. You'll see.

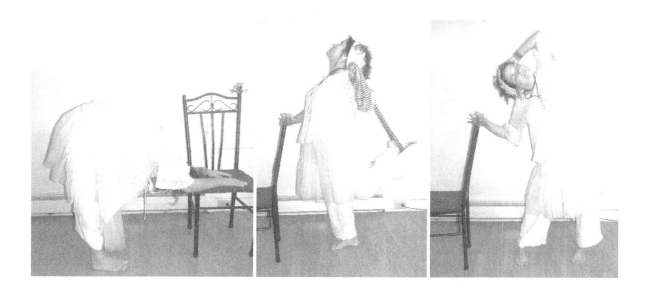

ROLL DOWN (BL)

Affirmation:
    I recover vibrant health and strong bones.

Legs close; toes in.
Roll down slowly.
Breathe 2 or 3 times at each pause.
Pause to stretch -back of neck
            -back of shoulders
                -middle back
                -lower back
                -buttocks
                -back of legs
Shift weight to the left foot
Shift weight to the right foot
Roll up slowly to stand

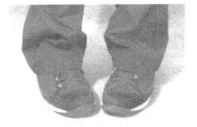

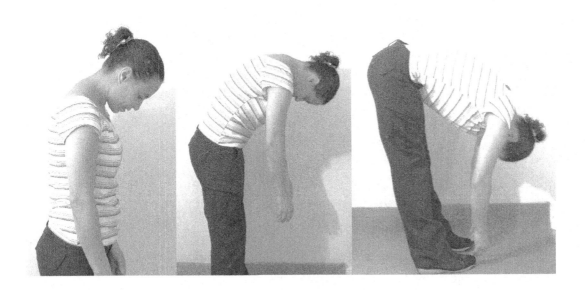

SQUEEZE THE KIDNEYS (KI)

Affirmation:
   I welcome vitality and stamina.

Feet wide; toes out
Hips forward (stretch inner thigh)
Shift weight to left leg. Breath
Shift weight to right leg. Breath
Return to center
Feet wide; toes forward (sit or hold chair for balance if needed)
Arch head back (stretch neck)
Arch your back (stretch the abdomen)
Breathe 2 or 3 times.

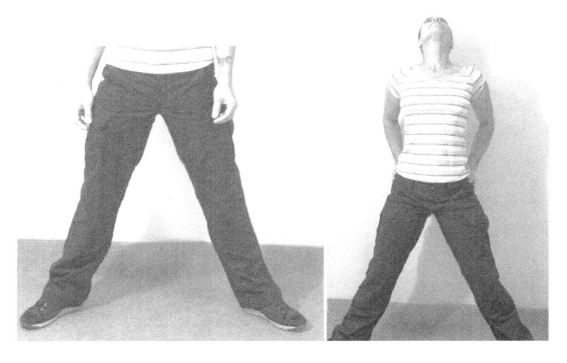

LIFT THE HEART (PC)

Affirmation:
My heart is strengthened and protected.

Feet wide; toes forward (or sit in chair)
Spread arms and fingers wide
Wrists back (stretch at wrist and elbow)
Squeeze shoulder blades together.
Breathe 2 or 3 times.

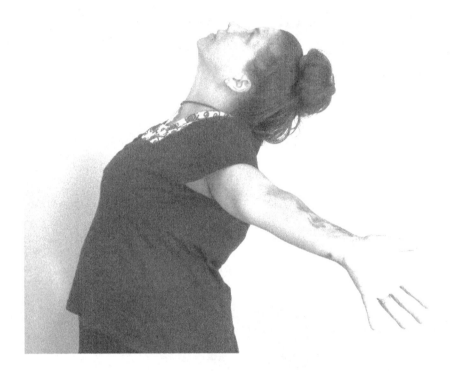

CURL THE ARM (TH)

Affirmation:

My immune system is strong. I feel serene.

Feet wide; toes forward
Make a fist with your left hand
Place fist under right clavicle
Use right hand to pull left elbow toward center.
    (stretch back of wrist and back of shoulder)
Drop head to the right, ear to sky (stretch neck).
Breathe 2 or 3 times.
Return to center
Repeat for the other side

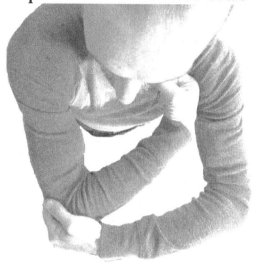 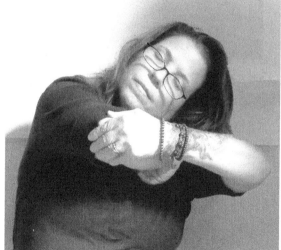

SIDE BODY (GB)

Affirmation:
    I am flexible and balanced.

Feet wide; toes in
Bend right knee; left hand behind back
Lean head right (stretch neck)
Lean torso right (stretch hip)
Raise left arm overhead (stretch side torso). Breathe 3 to 5 times.
Return to center
Repeat for the other side

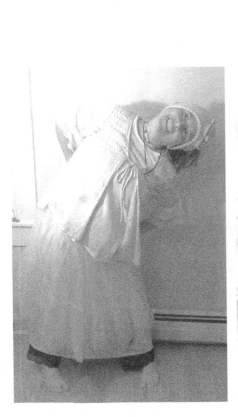
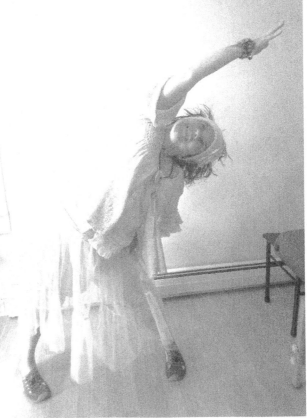

LIFT THE LIVER (LV)

Affirmation:
  I release all anger, tension and frustration.

Feet wide, toes out
Hips forward (stretch inner knee)
Arch back, ribs to the sky (stretch abdomen)
Lean to the right (stretch side abdomen). Breathe 2 or 3 times.
Return to center
Repeat for other side

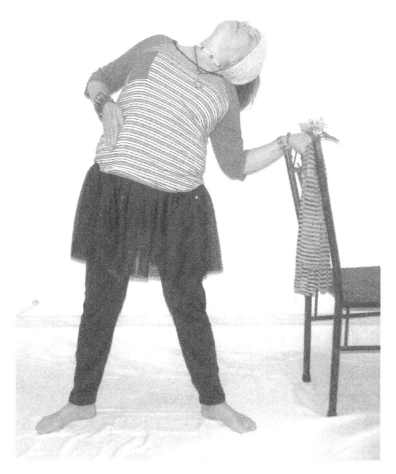

SHOULDER OPENER (LU)

Affirmation:
   I release all grief, and welcome inspiration.

Feet wide, toes forward
Press shoulders down, neck long, elbows straight
Flex your wrists, palms down and thumbs pointing back
Glide your shoulders back to open the chest. Breathe 2 or 3 times.

Alternative
Interlace your fingers, palms <u>down</u>
Straighten elbows (stretch wrists)
Shoulders down and back (stretch shoulders)

If you can do prayer hands behind your back, you win!
(again, shoulders down and back)

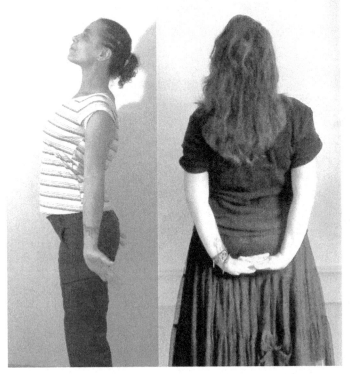
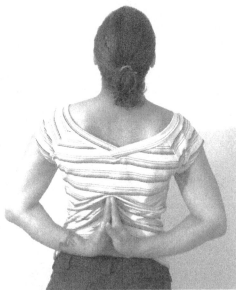

NECK AND SHOULDER RELEASE (LI)

Affirmation:
　　I let go of everything that is a detriment.

Feet wide; toes forward
Interlace fingers, palms <u>up</u> (stretch shoulders)
Straighten elbows (stretch wrists)
Drop head to the left, nose to sky (stretch neck)
Breathe 2 or 3 times.
Return to center
Repeat for the other side

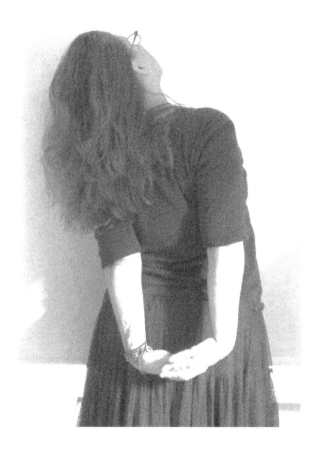

DOLPHIN STRETCH (ST)

Affirmation:

I accept nourishment, information and support.

Bend left knee

Grasp left foot with hand or scarf (stretch quads)

Pull knee back (stretch front of hip)

Arch back (stretch abdomen)

Head back (stretch neck) Breathe 2 or 3 times.

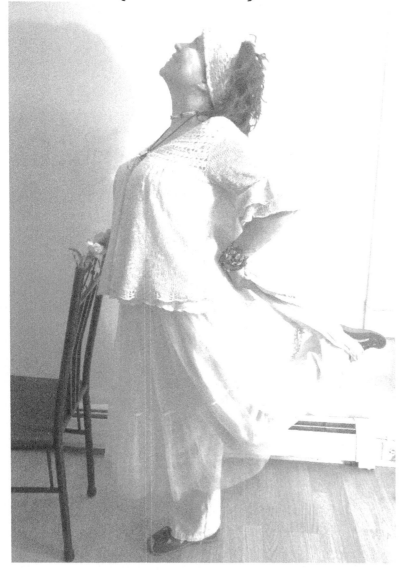

RELAX IN THE GRASS (SP)

Affirmation:
   I skillfully process and transform all my experiences.

Feet close, toes in, hips forward
Lace hands on the head
Arch back (stretch abdomen)
Lean Right (stretch side torso).
Breathe 2 or 3 times.
Return to center
Repeat on other side

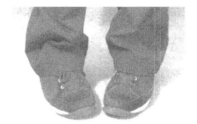

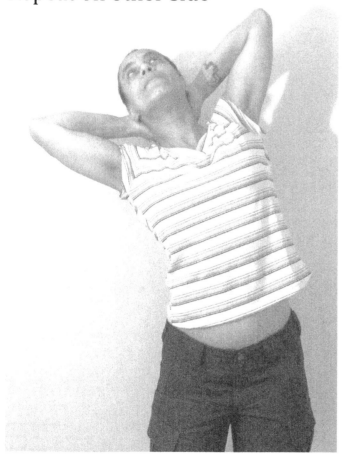

REACH FOR HEAVEN (HT)

Affirmation:
   I love myself and welcome all that is divine.

Interlace fingers, palms to sky
Shoulders down (do not shrug)
Straighten elbows
Look up
Lean slightly back. Breathe 2 or 3 times.

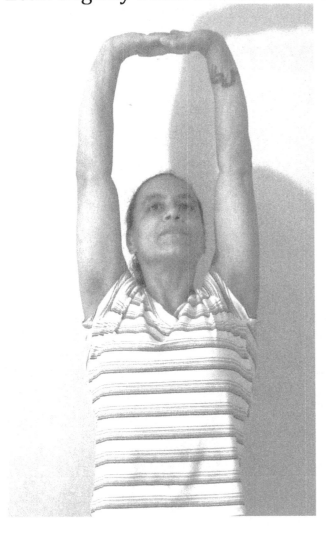

SELF HUG (SI)

Affirmation:

I am selective about what I allow into my life.

Left hand on right shoulder
Use right arm to pull left elbow closer
Lean left, ear to the sky. Breathe 2 or 3 times.
Return to center
Repeat for the other side

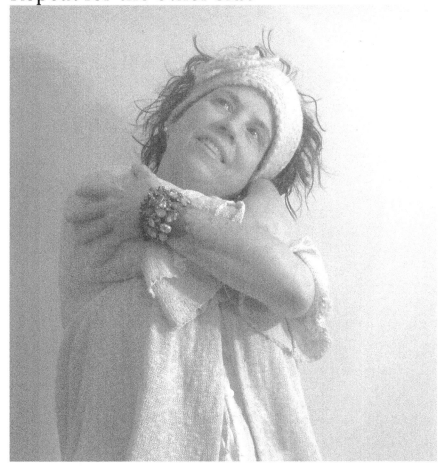

SHAKE IT OFF

Affirmation:
    All that has been released, is removed.

Shake and jostle every part of your body
Bounce and jiggle your entire body
(to release stress and increase lymph circulation)

Don't you feel great now?

WEEKEND SERIES QUICK LIST

ROLL DOWN (BL)
  – I recover vibrant health and strong bones.

SQUEEZE THE KIDNEYS (KI)
  – I welcome vitality and stamina.

LIFT THE HEART (PC)
  – My heart is strengthened and protected.

CURL THE ARM (TH)
  – My immune system is strong
      and my outward expression is serene.

SIDE BODY (GB)
  – I am flexible and balanced.

LIFT THE LIVER (LV)
  – I release all anger, tension and frustration.

SHOULDER OPENER (LU)
  – I release all grief, and welcome inspiration.

NECK AND SHOULDER RELEASE (LI)
  – I radically let go of everything which is a detriment.

DOLPHIN STRETCH (ST)
  – I accept nourishment, information and support.

RELAX IN THE GRASS (SP)
  – I skillfully process and transform all my experiences.

REACH FOR HEAVEN (HT)
  - I love myself and welcome all that is Divine.

SELF HUG (SI)
  - I am selective about what I allow into my life.

SHAKE IT OFF
  - All that has been released, is now removed.

Keep it moving.   I wish you well.

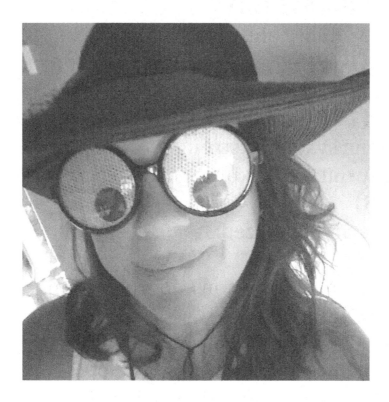

RESOURCES

Archer, Pat. Nelson, Lisa (2013) *Applied Anatomy &Physiology for Manual Therapists.*

Werner, Ruth. (2016) *A Massage Therapist's Guide to Pathology, Critical Thinking and Practical Application.*

Moorcroft, Cindy, LMT (2011) *Myology and Kinesiology for Massage Therapists*

McGreevy, M., Crinnin, M. Alexander, D. (2012) *Shiatsu Workbook*

Mattes, Aaron (2000) *Active Isolated Stretching: The Mattes Method*

Biel, Andrew (2014) *Trail Guide to the Body: A hands-on guide to locating muscles, bones and more.*

Biel, Andrew (2015) *Trial Guide to Movement: Building the Body in Motion*

Nelson, Marilee (2015). *Lymph: The Missing Link in Liver Detox.* Retrieved from
https://branchbasics.com/blog/2015/09/16-ways-to-activate-your-lymphatic-system

Ellis, Wiseman, Boss and Cleaver (2004) *Fundamentals of Chinese Acupuncture*

Beaulieu, T. (2017, November). *Thought Field Therapy.* Workshop based upon the book Fit for Love;
manifest, understand and transform your blueprint presented at Mettabee Farm in Harlemville, NY.

ABOUT THE AUTHOR

Bleu Andersen is a Licensed Massage Therapist, collage-maker, motorcyclist,
mender, photographer, artist, Facebook Addict,
and a writer of bad poetry with a wee bit of a Superman complex.
She possesses an active mind and sensitive soul being hindered by a human body
experiencing the illusion of mortality while learning about the infinite universe
through a 3-dimentional filter.

Made in the USA
Middletown, DE
21 February 2020